ARE YOU HAVING FUN?

Doing All the Things You Want to Do?

CAROL CHESHIRE

iUniverse, Inc.
Bloomington

Are You Having Fun?
Doing All the Things You Want to Do?

iUniverse books may be ordered through booksellers or by contacting:

iUniverse
1663 Liberty Drive
Bloomington, IN 47403
www.iuniverse.com
1-800-Authors (1-800-288-4677)

ISBN: 978-1-4620-1798-0 (sc)
ISBN: 978-1-4620-1796-6 (e)

Library of Congress Control Number: 2011906888

Printed in the United States of America

iUniverse rev. date: 04/29/2011

This book was written with the help of Donna Kozik.

*My sister-in-law was a great stimulus
to me to accomplish this book.*

ARE YOU
HAVING
FUN?

Doing All the Things
You Want to Do?

Carol grew up in Houston, Texas. She taught school when it was not as it is today.

The schools' were good in preparing their students. Carol taught school for several years, in good districts east of Houston.

Carol got her degrees from the University of Houston at Clear Lake. She received a BS and a MS degree. During this time, she had to take several classes to fulfill requirements for different certifications in her field. When teaching, counseling is a big part of the job.

Carol moved to Central Texas when she retired. She lives on 20 acres with trees and wildlife as well as her dog, Cocoa.

Carol took a psychology class that would certify her to be able to counsel people of all ages. Then, she counseled several local people with various problems.

She has since done marketing on the computer. The one job that stands out most is the Founders Membership in Tobri.com.

You can contact her at lapixit9@ gmail.com

This book has been a huge introduction on where to go and how to solve my teenage son's addictions and family problems.

Thank, Carol, you mean a lot to me.

Contents

ILL Habits gather by unseen degrees.
As brooks make rivers, rivers run to seas.

~John Dryden, *Absalom and Achitophel*, 1681

Bad habits are easier to abandon today than tomorrow.

~Yiddish Proverb

1

We are born develop-ing habits. There is an incident of an Ultra Sound on a pregnant woman that showed the Fetus sucking its' thumb. This illustrated an early habit of sucking. Babies cry when they want to be changed or fed. This also is a developed habit illustrated by the parents rewarding them by 1) making them more comfortable 2) giving them attention and affection. Habits repeated over a period of time can easily become an addiction. (Wood W. Neal DT) (2007). "A new look at habits and the habit goal-interface." Psychological Review.1142 843-863 Addiction can be defined as two aspects: substance addiction and process addictions. Substance addictions include alcohol, illegal drugs, prescription drug and nicotine. A process addiction is defined as an addiction to an action such as gambling, shopping, working, sexual activities, eating and cleaning. All of which can come from habitual repetition over time.

Addiction can manifest as physical or mental dependency. Regardless of the addiction there are common factors in substance or process addictions.

An actual craving, physical need or uncontrolled desire for a substance or an action is physical dependency. Substances and some actions change the body chemistry of the individual, so that the body thinks it needs the substance or activity to survive. Withdrawal begins when the body does not get the desired stimulus. Withdrawal can be mild or lead to death threatening reactions, depending on the stimulus .It depends on the type of stimulus as well as the length of time it has been used.

A mental dependency is when an individual feels they have a need for the stimulus to get through the day or a situation. Addiction can be physical, mental or a combination of the two.

There are many factors in addictions, since it can begin before birth. Most are not ever thought of as addictions such as: brushing teeth, washing hands, dressing following the usual rituals to go about a normal day and normal lives.

Habit is a second nature which prevents us from knowing the first, of which it has neither cruelties nor the enchantments.

~Marcel Proust

There are several definitions for addiction: such as addictive personality-an aspect of a persons' fundamental personality or character. This can be illustrated by compulsive hand washing, fear of heights, and phobias too numerous to mention.

Addiction to an action or routine of actions is a good illustration of the behavior. Such as gambling, over eating or not eating, shopping for things you do not need, over working or sexual activities. Acquiring or participating in addictive movement or process; that can lead to acquiring these addictions.

When regular use of a drug, alcohol, or other substances build up within the users' body; the body becomes accustomed to the substance, thus higher levels or desired to reach the effect the user desires.

It is believed some people are predisposed genetically to developing an addiction. (Plotnik, 1999).Supposedly the individual's body chemistry is such they are sensitive to drugs, alcohol, and other substances making them more vulnerable to addiction.

Social learning is considered an important factor in addictions. In family environments where this action is indulged in may lead to this belief. (Laland K.N. and G.R. Brown, 2002). Another big area, peer pressure, advertising or media maybe a big influence on users. Some use substances to help vent stress. Many can be violent through their venting.

There is an old saying, author unknown, "Monkey see Monkey do."

This seems to fit many individuals first starting out developing a habit or addiction.

Socially immature individuals, such as teenagers looking for acceptance by their peers, will develop the acceptable habits within the group. They make decisions based on the behaviors of stronger willed peers.

Habits are formed from learning and beliefs. Once a habit is formed, most of the time it is difficult to make a change. ~ As Samuel Johnson said,

> *"the chains of habit are generally too small to be felt until they are too strong to be broken".*

> *Small habits well pursued betimes*
> *May reach the dignity of crimes.*
>
> ~Hannah More

> *A habit is something you do without thinking-which is why most of us have so many of them.*
>
> ~Frank A. Clark

2

Many scientists feel that the use of behavior modification is the sole success story for controlling and stopping addiction of any kind.

Behavior modification is a term that often appears in magazine articles describing research in changing people's behavior through drugs, "mind control", or even brain surgery. In fact, it is none of these things. They refer to behavior modification as learning principles (classical conditioning, operant conditioning and social learning) to change people's actions and feelings. (See Pavlov, studies on classical conditioning.)

Behavior modification involves a series of well-defined steps to change behavior. The success of each step is carefully evaluated to find the best solution for a given situation.

One theory of behavior modification is the use of a token economy. This is a reward system for desired behavior. In classroom situations this may work for a short period. For example, as long as a reward is given for the desired behavior, the effects are usually positive.

It was thought that the student would slowly change when the token was removed on a scheduled basis. It is rarely a long term solution, however, because many students as well as adults always require some type of token for desired behavior. (Cohen and Filipczak,1971).

When a disruptive student makes teaching an impossible task and when normal disciplinary actions fail, they are usually referred to a psychologist. They are, (many may say often times, to harsh and inappropriate) usually prescribed a drug to alter their behavior. Basically, a child with attention deficit hyperactive disorder, can, and will be prescribed medications such as Ritalin and Adderall. In truth, many studies say that this is just a quick fix for the student, parents and teachers. (NINDS Attention Deficit- Hyper Activity Disorder Information Page. National Institute of Neurological Disorders and Stroke (NINDS/NIH) February 2007.

3

In a case study of a drug abuser it would work only as long as they were in a controlled environment. When they returned to their normal environment the drug habit would return. Most treatment centers hold those who enter into treatment for three to six-weeks. Instead, it was found that the user reverted to use of the substance after this short amount of time. Removing the user from the environment for at least a year was found to keep the user clean. Some however, put back in the same environment with the same associates would revert back to their habit.

It is recommended for those individuals to be removed from their environment and social group for a year. (Seligman, Martin, E. F Walker, D.L. Rosenhanin *Abnormal Psychology,* 2000) Activities that keep their minds occupied and busy help a great deal. More activities should be used to develop self-control.

Let me stop at this point, to point out an individual must conclude they have a bad habit and desire change. If they refuse to admit they have a problem there is nothing anyone can do. Knowing the risks they are taking and a potential deadly outcome seems to elude their thinking. Most addicts know they have a problem, but do not think anything negative will ever happen to them because of their use of whatever substance they use.

Another case study that was handled concerned a young man: who called about 2AM in the morning to get help. He was sitting in a bath tub with water and a hair dryer in his hand. He had decided his life was not worth living. He was a drug user and was high and alone. After 2 hours of talking, someone managed to get to him. (Cheshire, Carolyn, 1989).After this he was admitted for treatment and went home to his family.

Tobacco is one of the most difficult habits to change. It also falls under behavior modification. To become a non-tobacco user is as hard as becoming a non-drug user.

There have been several substitutes for tobacco use developed in the last few years. However, they are only temporary stop gaps for users. Some examples include the patch, gum, and lozenges.

People have been using tobacco since before Europeans discovered North and South America. Indigenous peoples, already addicted to the locally grown plant, shared their source of "calm and peace" with the newcomers. Tobacco use, ranging from snuff, to pipes, to the later, more convenient form of cigarettes spread across Europe and the world.

Since tobacco use became unacceptable and scientifically proven to cause deadly diseases such as COPD and cancer, many scientists have searched for a way to help tobacco addicts stop use of the drug. (Nichterm, Cartwright,1991). Most users claim someone they were close to did it so; why should I worry it is probably not in my genes. They wager their life for a drug fix. This is before breakfast, after breakfast, on the way to work, on any break during the day, on their way home, after dinner or a drink or two, before they go to bed and if they cannot sleep another is indulged in. Some fall asleep smoking causing fire that can kill them.

These "specialists" who tried to help tobacco addicts quit the habit first declared people could just quit--in other words, go "cold turkey". People found that more than 90% who tried this method, returned (as other drug users) to use of the product. There have been modification methods such as a change of where people smoked, shock therapy, shock therapy, sitting in a closed room with other smokers forced to smoke a carton of cigarettes (called aversion therapy). All of these methods have failed for the most part.

In the past 4-5 years, specialists are using the Electronic cigarette. As the sister-in-law of a tobacco addict, she has pleased the entire family from a gradual slowdown of nicotine use. The "cigarette" (with the tar and carbon monoxide left out) has tremendously helped thousands of people by the use of this product. It seems to have the practical use of behavior modification by providing a drop of nicotine, the "puff" and something to hold. It seems that an "e-cigarette" user does not offend persons in an area near them. There is no second hand smoke. Many advertisers say e-cigarettes are not for smoking termination; however thousands of smokers have been able to kick the habit. Every person I know who has been successful with the e-cigarette is very proud of themselves. This is a very important experience for the former addict as it will help them not return to the use of the real habit of smoking this may be the way of the future for current smokers to find a solution for an addiction. As negative habits become positive,

Habit is cable; we weave a thread each day and at last we cannot break it.

~Horace Mann

4

Definition of modeling: learning by imitating others; copying behavior.

"A study of TV and Violence was released in 1996 by Mediascope. They found by watching violence on television, viewers risk the following results: (1)They learn to behave violently. (2) They become more desensitized to violence. (3) They become more fearful of being attacked."

Can you imagine how they feel today with the movies becoming more and more violent. Little children cannot even laugh at comics because they are monsters, vampires, super weird heroes.

Modeling basically is divided into three parts and includes three different types of effects. The simplest case-the first type of modeling-is the behavior patterns of others. Simply this increases the chances that they will do the same things, the same way. Examples are they clap when others do, look up at a building if everyone else does and copy styles and verbal expressions of peers.

The second type is usually called observational learning, or imitation. An observer watches someone perform the behavior, thus being able then to copy the behavior. Some can distinguish the difference between good and bad. Others cannot.

The latest children's movies deal with wizards, vampires and werewolves. These characters appear to be a good versus evil. Their representation can only be false because of the very idea.

A third type of modeling involves inhibition or the lack of. When an observer watches threatening activity without being a punishment, the observer may find it easier to engage in the behavior later. An example might be seeing someone steal something and not be punished. They then think hey that was easy, why not just do it.

Today's society makes this type off modeling a breeze for the imitators to imitate the behaviors they want to have.

5

Habit is a man's sole comfort. We dislike doing without even unpleasant things to which we have become accustomed.

~Goethe

Society and peers put the pressure on the individual to participate in order to be accepted. Few can withstand this pressure.

Entertainers, athletes and television put the same pressure as the peer group. They make undesirable habits look enchanting and the way to go. To be the in group, follow their lead. In other words follow me and be a real leader, be the star.

Self-control has all but gone out the window. People have to set up personal goals to defeat societal pressures. Without self-control we are a wandering soul looking for any means to soothe our yens.

People acquire certain behaviors through classical conditioning, a learning procedure in which associations are made between a neutral stimulus and a conditional response, differently to dissimilar stimuli.

> *Enduring habits I hate...Yes, at the very bottom of my soul I feel grateful to all my misery and bouts of sickness and everything about me that is imperfect, because this sort of thing leaves me with a hundred back doors through which I can escape from enduring habits.*
>
> ~ Friedrich Nietzsche, 1982

Most of life is habitual. We do the same things we did yesterday, the day before and every day for life. Estimates indicate that out of our conscious process, we get 40 out of 11,000 signals our brain produces.

To effect change in habits, one needs to bring the action back into the ability to make choices. Change is hard work and there is no shortcut to achieve this goal. The first step in breaking a bad habit is to determine what makes it so desirable. What negative thing compels us? What could be the positive effect? We've weighed the choices-what are the tradeoffs-we must make a choice now to read this book is a conscious choice.

The whole reason we form habits in the first place is to fill a need. As we break the old pattern we still need to fulfill that need. We will not only be ridding ourselves of negative habits, it will also be making a choice to better perform a better alternative. The choice lies in what you decide to replace bad habits with.

There are so many habits you could have a dictionary of nothing but human habits.

Habit with him was all the test of truth;
It must be right: I've done it from my youth.

~George Crabbe, *The Borough*

Habits good or bad make you who you are. Changing your habits, even a small amount can create a change in you.

If you find a need for counseling contact Carol at lapixit9@gmail.com and she will give you a phone number by which she can be reached.

She can be reached on TOBRI.com as well.

Inside you will find the different kinds of habits we each have lurking in our lives.

Some points are made to possible solutions and cures.

NOTES

NOTES

NOTES

NOTES

NOTES

NOTES

NOTES

NOTES

NOTES

NOTES

NOTES

NOTES

www.ingramcontent.com/pod-product-compliance
Lightning Source LLC
Chambersburg PA
CBHW061228280526
45784CB00006B/2686